How to overcome low sperm count

Conquering male infertility

Refuge Victor

All rights reserved. No part of this publication may be reproduced, distributed, or transmitted in any form or by any means, including photocopying, recording, or other electronic or mechanical methods, without the prior written permission of the publisher, except in the case of brief quotations embodied to critical reviews and certain other noncommercial uses permitted by copyright law.

Copyright © Refuge Victor, 2023

Table of content

Chapter One
What low sperm count is all about

A low sperm count, likewise called oligozoospermia, is where a man has less than 15 million sperm for each milliliter of semen.

Having a low sperm count can make it more challenging to consider normally, albeit effective pregnancies can in any case happen.

Issues with sperm, including a low sperm count and issues with sperm quality, are very normal. They're a figure around 1 of every 3 couples who are attempting to get pregnant.

There are medicines accessible on the NHS or secretly that can assist you with becoming a father assuming you have a low sperm count.

Getting your sperm count checked
See your GP if you have not figured out how to consider following 1 year of pursuing a child.

It's smart for both you and your accomplice to get guidance, as richness issues can influence people and frequently it's a blend of both. It's essential to comprehend what the specific issue is before you settle on your following stages.

One of the tests your GP can organize is a semen investigation.

This is where an example of semen is examined to look at the quality and amount of the sperm. The outcomes are generally accessible soon.

On the off chance that the outcomes are not ordinary, the test ought to be rehashed to guarantee it was exact. This will regularly be performed following 3 months.

Your GP can refer you to an expert in male barrenness at your neighborhood medical clinic or fruitfulness facility if any issues are found.

Home sperm count testing units
There are a few male fruitfulness home-testing units accessible to purchase from drug stores. These tests guarantee to show whether your sperm count is low.

It could be enticing to attempt one of the tests if you would prefer not to see your GP, yet you ought to know that:

Even though exploration by the producers recommends these tests can give a precise sign of sperm count, they have not been widely considered

Some home-testing packs characterize a low sperm considered under 20 million sperm for each milliliter of semen, however later worldwide rules express that anything over 15 million sperm for every milliliter of semen is ordinary

A few units take a look at the quantity of sperm, rather than different things that can influence richness, for example, how well the sperm can not do the work move (motility) - utilizing a pack that actions both these things is ideal

While these tests could give a valuable sign of your sperm count, they may likewise give you bogus consolation or may propose your sperm count is low when it's very considered common.

It's smarter to see your GP for a legitimate semen examination at a certified research center if you're worried about your fruitfulness. Perceive how to utilize individual test units securely for additional about the issues of home testing.

Ripeness specialists consider sperm count a significant element for fruitfulness. Approaches to helping sperm count range from getting more rest and stopping smoking to dietary changes and medicine.

Sperm count alludes to the typical number of sperm present in one example of semen. In light of the latest World Wellbeing Association (WHO) rules, specialists consider an energizing sperm build-up to be 15 million for every milliliter (ml), or if nothing else 39 million for each discharge.

Specialists consider a sperm count under 15 million for each ml to be low, and it might cause fruitfulness issues.

By and large, well-being experts accept that factors that impact testosterone levels essentially affect sperm number and quality.
Counting acquired hereditary problems, contaminations, and growths can likewise influence sperm count.

Notwithstanding, a few way-of-life decisions and regular cures can assist with supporting the chemicals that control sperm creation, which might help the sound improvement of sperm and further develop sperm count.
For quite some time, scientists have realized that sperm quality and richness rates have been declining in most Western countries.

As per one 2017 review, the typical sperm include in North America, Europe, Australia, and New Zealand dropped by 59.3% somewhere in the range between 1973 and 2011.
Despite studies having distinguished this, researchers don't completely grasp the purpose behind this downfall. Investigation into dependable techniques for switching a low sperm count is continuous.

Chapter Two
Causes of low sperm count

A man has a few numbers that act as signs of good well-being: cholesterol, pulse, and weight/BMI to give some examples. At the point when you see a TFC male fruitfulness-trained professional, you will likewise add one more: sperm count.

What the vast majority allude to as a sperm count is a sperm focus, as it addresses the quantity of sperm present in one milliliter (mL) of semen. A standard semen examination (or sperm test) gauges three essential variables: sperm fixation, sperm motility (or the percent of sperm that are effectively swimming), and sperm morphology (shape).

An ordinary sperm fixation is something like 20 million for each mL, while typical motility is no less than half and typical morphology is no less than 15%. While there are numerous other significant elements engaged with a semen investigation - like fundamental volume, the presence or nonattendance of white platelets, and the nature of sperm development (to give some examples), most laypeople center around sperm focus.

If a semen examination uncovers a low sperm count, we will play out extra testing to determine the reason.
A few cases might warrant a reference to a male urologist richness, and we work with the best ones in Focal Texas. It might urge you to realize that through our cooperative methodology, TFC can effectively treat virtually all instances of male component fruitlessness. A few cases can be treated with mina or way of life changes, while others might require a prescription, medical procedure, or lab help with the type of either intrauterine insemination (IUI) or in vitro preparation (IVF). Notwithstanding, there is an amazing visualization for essentially all men who seek treatment.

Reasons for low sperm count

Medical procedures, Diseases, Momentum and Past Medical problems

Mumps, physically communicated sicknesses like Chlamydia or urinary lot diseases can leave scars that block the sensitive cylinders that transport sperm from the testicles to the penis. Spinal rope wounds, diabetes, and certain medical procedures can impede the typical progression of sperm, or potentially lead to retrograde (in reverse) discharge.

Hereditary or Persistent Infection
While most hereditary reasons for low or the total shortfall of sperm creation are interesting, numerous constant circumstances or potential meds used to treat them are normal reasons for male fruitlessness. Conditions, for example, malignant growth of the gonad or prostate, diabetes, hypertension, and fringe vascular illness can make a man have a low sperm count.

Lifesaving malignant growth therapy either medical procedure, chemotherapy, or radiation treatment can obliterate sperm cells, and incredibly decline a man's sperm count. TFC offers fruitfulness salvage preceding disease treatment to proactively safeguard future ripeness.

Primary Issues with the Penis or Gonads
Primary issues with the penis that can cause a man's sperm to build up to fall incorporate Peyronie's illness (in which plaque or potentially scar tissue develops in the penis), as well as issues with irritation and scar tissue that can obstruct the typical ejaculatory process. A varicocele is available in up to 40 percent of men with fruitfulness issues and is a condition that can once in a while influence ripeness. While most men with a varicocele won't need or profit from a medical procedure, the condition warrants a discussion with a fruitfulness subject matter expert.

Other possibly significant underlying issues incorporate undescended balls, sperm channel issues, and blockages in the cylinders that transport sperm (vas deferens).

Hormonal Awkward nature

Chemicals drive the creation of sperm, and some of the time the hormonal signs between the mind, pituitary, and balls can slow down or stop out and out. A blood test can affirm whether all frameworks are working, or on the other hand on the off chance that a lopsidedness is causing a low sperm count.

Past Vasectomy
Medical procedures to switch vasectomy can deliver success in reestablishing patency in the cylinders that convey sperm. The results of the medical procedure, notwithstanding, may lead a man to create antibodies that can go after his sperm.

Drugs for Low T
Get some information about the drugs that might prompt a low sperm count, including famous Low T treatments. Men who have been involved in anabolic steroids for expanded timeframes may encounter a low sperm count as an outcome. Generally speaking, these incidental effects are transitory, and ripeness is reestablished after essentially halting the medicine.

Natural and Way of Life Elements
Certain propensities and occupations put men in danger for fruitfulness issues, and a lower sperm count can make it challenging to become a dad. Embrace a refreshing way of life and weight while attempting to consider, and you will expand your opportunities for progress. The most well-known dangers to a man's richness include:

- Liquor misuse
- Anabolic steroids
- Cigarette smoking
- Openness to harmful synthetic substances, weighty metals, pesticides, paint and solvents
- Unlawful medications, including cocaine and marijuana
- Weight

In outrageous cases, delayed openness to warm and significant distance cycling can likewise influence a man's fruitfulness and leave him with a low sperm count. In these cases, a difference in propensities might be the main essential strategy.

Indications of low sperm count
- The failure to consider normally (no female fruitfulness issue present)
- Sexual brokenness (low drive, erectile brokenness)
- Testicular anomalies (torment/inconvenience, lump(s), or enlarging)
- Proof of a hormonal or chromosomal issue (loss of body/beard growth)

On the off chance that any of the above side effects are available, a visit to a doctor is prescribed to get a finding and start a treatment plan.

Chapter Three
Diagnosis and treatment for low sperm count

At the point when you see a specialist since you're experiencing difficulty getting your accomplice pregnant, the individual in question will attempt to decide the basic reason. Regardless of whether your PCP thinks low sperm count is the issue, it is prescribed that your accomplice be assessed to preclude possible contributing variables and decide whether helped conceptive procedures might be required.

General actual assessment and clinical history

This incorporates assessment of your private parts and posing inquiries about any acquired circumstances, constant medical conditions, sicknesses, wounds, or medical procedures that could influence fruitfulness. Your primary care physician could likewise get some information about your sexual propensities and your sexual turn of events.

Semen examination

A low sperm consider is analyzed piece of a semen examination test. Sperm count is not set in stone by looking at semen under a magnifying lens to perceive the number of sperm that show up inside squares on a lattice design. At times, a PC may be utilized to gauge sperm count.

Semen tests can be obtained in two or three distinct ways. You can give an example by stroking off and discharging into a unique holder at the specialist's office. Due to strict or social convictions, a few men favor an elective strategy for semen assortment. In such cases, semen can be gathered by utilizing an extraordinary condom during intercourse.

New sperm are delivered constantly in the gonads and take around 42 to 76 days to develop. Thus, an ongoing semen examination mirrors your current circumstances throughout recent months. Any sure switches you've made won't show around for a very long time.

One of the most widely recognized reasons for low sperm count is a fragmented or inappropriate assortment of sperm tests. Sperm counts additionally frequently vary. In light of these elements, most specialists will check at least two semen tests over the long run to guarantee consistency between tests.

To guarantee exactness in an assortment, your PCP will:

- Request that you ensure all of your semen makes it into the assortment cup or assortment condom when you discharge
- Have you gone without discharging for two to seven days before gathering an example
- Gather a second example something like fourteen days after the first
- Have you stayed away from the utilization of oils because these items can influence sperm motility
- Semen investigation results

Typical sperm densities range from 15 million to more noteworthy than 200 million sperm for every milliliter of semen. You are considered to have a low sperm count on the off chance that you have less than 15 million sperm for every milliliter or under 39 million sperm all out per discharge.

Your possibility of getting your accomplice pregnant reduces with diminishing sperm counts. A few men have no sperm in their semen by any means. This is known as azoospermia (ay-zoh-uh-Spike me-uh).

There are many variables engaged with multiplication, and the quantity of sperm in your semen is only one. A few men with low sperm counts effectively father kids. Similarly, a few men with ordinary sperm counts can't father youngsters. Regardless of whether you have sufficient sperm, different elements are critical to accomplish a pregnancy, including ordinary sperm development (motility).

Contingent upon starting discoveries, your primary care physician could prescribe extra tests to search for the reason for your low sperm count and other potential reasons for male barrenness. These can include:

Scrotal ultrasound. This test utilizes high-recurrence sound waves to check out the balls and supporting designs.

Chemical testing. Your PCP could prescribe a blood test to decide the degree of chemicals created by the pituitary organ and gonads, which assume a vital part in the sexual turn of events and sperm creation.

Post-discharge urinalysis. Sperm in your pee can show your sperm are voyaging in reverse into the bladder rather than out your penis during discharge (retrograde discharge).

Hereditary tests. At the point when sperm fixation is very low, hereditary causes could be involved. A blood test can uncover whether there are unobtrusive changes in the Y chromosome — indications of a hereditary irregularity. Hereditary testing could likewise be requested to analyze different inherent or acquired conditions.

Testicular biopsy. This test includes eliminating tests from the gonad with a needle. The consequences of the testicular biopsy can figure out whether sperm creation is typical. On the off chance that it is, your concern is reasonably brought about by a blockage or one more issue with sperm transport. Be that as it may, this test is normally just utilized in specific circumstances and isn't usually used to analyze the reason for fruitlessness.

Hostile to sperm neutralizer tests. These tests, which are utilized to check for safe cells (antibodies) that assault sperm and influence their capacity to work, are not normal.

Particular sperm capability tests. Various tests can be utilized to check how well your sperm get by after discharge, how well they can enter an egg, and whether there's any issue connecting to the egg. These tests are seldom performed and frequently don't fundamentally change treatment proposals.

Transrectal ultrasound. A little greased-up wand is embedded into your rectum to take a look at your prostate and check for blockages of the cylinders that convey semen (ejaculatory conduits and original vesicles).

Medicines for low sperm count include:

Medical procedure. For instance, a varicocele can frequently be precisely remedied or a hindered vas deferens can be fixed. Earlier vasectomies can be turned around. In situations where no sperm is available in the discharge, sperm can frequently be recovered straightforwardly from the balls or epididymis utilizing sperm recovery methods.

Treating contaminations. Anti-microbials can fix a disease of the regenerative parcel, yet this doesn't necessarily in every case reestablish fruitfulness.

Medicines for sex issues. Prescription or directing can assist with further developing fruitfulness in conditions like erectile brokenness or untimely discharge.

Chemical medicines and prescriptions. Your PCP could suggest chemical substitution or prescriptions in situations where fruitlessness is brought about by high or low levels of specific chemicals or issues with how the body utilizes chemicals.

Helped conceptive innovation (Craftsmanship). Workmanship medicines include getting sperm through typical discharge, careful extraction, or from contributor people, contingent upon your particular circumstance and wishes. The sperm are then embedded into the female genital lot, or utilized for IVF or intracytoplasmic sperm infusion.

At the point when treatment doesn't work

In uncommon cases, male richness issues can't be dealt with, and it's unimaginable for a man to father a kid. If so, you and your accomplice can consider either utilizing sperm from a contributor or embracing a kid.

Chapter Four

Natural remedies for low sperm count

Specialists of old, natural, and customary medication have utilized a few nonpharmacologic solutions for increment sperm count and further development of sperm well-being for millennia. Furthermore, specialists have recommended that the vast majority of these cures can impact sperm somehow or another.

Coming up next are characteristic ways of expanding sperm count.

Get sufficient activity and rest

A few investigations have proposed that weight reduction and exercise among individuals with overweight or heft can prompt an improved or expanded sperm count. Nonetheless, the science of connecting a solid weight list (BMI) to a sound sperm count is as yet feeble.

Inspected the advantages of playing out a multi-week high-impact practice program of something like three 50-minute meetings each week. The members arrived at 50-65% of their pinnacle pulse.

In the review, standard activity expanded sperm and motility in 45 men with weight and stationary ways of life.

Stop smoking

A 2016 meta-examination that looked into the consequences of more than 20 investigations with a sum of almost 6,000 members found that smoking reliably decreased sperm count.

The scientists found that individuals who smoked moderate or weighty measures of tobacco had a lower sperm quality than individuals who smoked tobacco less intensely.

Keep away from extreme liquor and medication use

The number of controlled investigations to have investigated the connection between sperm well-being and medications is restricted. This is because testing unlawful substances can prompt moral issues.

Has connected the overall utilization of medications like liquor, cannabis, and cocaine to diminished sperm creation. Some proof is clashing, so further examination is important to affirm this connection.

Stay away from specific professionally prescribed meds

A few doctor-prescribed drugs might diminish sound sperm creation. When the male quits taking the medicine, in any case, their sperm count ought to get back to business as usual or increment.

Prescriptions that may briefly diminish the creation and advancement of sperm include:

- A few antimicrobials
- Enemies of androgens
- Hostile to inflammatories
- Antipsychotics
- Narcotics

- Antidepressants
- Anabolic steroids, which might keep on influencing sperm count for as long as 1 year after halting the drug
- Exogenous or strengthening testosterone
- Methadone

Guys ought to look for a conference with a medical services supplier on the off chance that they accept that a drug they are at present taking might be decreasing their sperm count or influencing their richness.

Take a fenugreek supplement

Fenugreek has for some time been used as a characteristic solution for unfortunate sperm well-being, and backers propose that it might assist with further developing sperm count.

Truth be told, one 2017 investigation discovered that the patent-forthcoming compound Furosap, which producers created from fenugreek seeds, altogether further developed generally speaking semen quality and sperm count.

Get sufficient vitamin D

Scientists are not completely certain why, but rather blood levels of vitamin D and calcium seem to affect sperm wellbeing.

Of 18 examinations, scientists tracked down a critical relationship between further developed ripeness in male members and a more elevated level of vitamin D in the blood.

Nonetheless, the review creators do prompt wariness when deciphering these outcomes, and they prescribe further clinical preliminaries to affirm their discoveries.

Research shows that a lack of calcium may likewise unfavorably influence sperm count.

Take ashwagandha

Ashwagandha, or Indian ginseng, has long had an impact on conventional drugs as a solution for a few types of sexual brokenness.

A recent report found that 46 guys with low sperm counts who required 675 milligrams of ashwagandha day to day for 90 days saw a 167% expansion in their sperm count.

Eat more cell reinforcement-rich food sources

Cancer prevention agents are particles that assist with deactivating intensifies called free revolutionaries, which harm cells.

A few nutrients and minerals go about as cell reinforcements and a few investigations have connected cell reinforcement utilization with expanded sperm count.

To a sound sperm count include:

- Beta-carotene
- Beta-cryptoxanthin
- Lutein
- L-ascorbic acid

Increment refreshing fat admission

Polyunsaturated fats are vital for the solid advancement of the sperm film. Such fats incorporate omega-3 and omega-6.

Three examinations found that guys with fruitlessness who enhanced with omega-3 unsaturated fats encountered a critical improvement in sperm motility and fixation, contrasted and guys who didn't take omega-3 enhancements.

Diminish unhealthful fat admission

A recent report reviewed 209 solid Spanish guys aged 18-23 years. The analysts found that as they expanded their utilization of trans unsaturated fats, their sperm count diminished proportionately.

Limit openness to natural and word-related pollutants

As contamination and clog increment, analysts frequently interface natural factors like air quality and openness to harmful synthetic substances to decrease sperm well-being and count.

Connected living in exceptionally modern regions with weighty air contamination to bring down sperm counts.

Keeping away from natural poisons as frequently as conceivable likewise adds to better general well-being.

Limit the utilization of soy and estrogen-rich food sources

A few food sources, particularly soy items, contain plant estrogen. This can decrease testosterone holding and sperm creation.

Of 1,319 guys in China found that higher convergences of plant estrogen in the semen implied lower quality sperm.

Many canned and plastic items are likewise high in engineered types of estrogen. Bisphenol A will be compounded to estrogen receptors in the body and may likewise influence male ripeness after openness, as per one 2019 survey.

Get sufficient folate and zinc

Restricted examinations propose that consuming folate and zinc in a blend might work on the general soundness of sperm, including focus and count.

Foods to improve sperm count

Generally, taking enhancements is a protected way for an individual to arrive at their everyday necessity for most nutrients, minerals, and cell reinforcements. Nonetheless, the body doesn't necessarily in all cases effectively retain them.

Most investigations propose that eating food varieties that give great measures of explicit mixtures and synthetic substances permits the body to effectively utilize them more.

The most ideal way to increment sperm count normally might be to build the utilization of food varieties high in sperm-accommodating supplements, like L-ascorbic acid, cancer prevention agents, and polyunsaturated fats.

Featured a few dietary examples that could prompt a low sperm count. These included:

- Eating high amounts of red and handled meat
- Not eating sufficient polyunsaturated unsaturated fat
- Having a high admission of energy
- Consuming low degrees of cancer prevention agents
- Consuming elevated degrees of immersed fats
- Eating restricted measures of foods grown from the ground.

No particular food is the way to expand sperm count through the eating regimen. All things considered, taking into account the eating routine is the most ideal way to further develop richness.

The survey did, nonetheless, feature melon as an especially strong food comparable to further developing sperm count.

A specialist might recommend medicine for guys with exceptionally low sperm counts and the video has extra well-being elements or contemplations.

Meds that specialists once in a while recommend to treat a low sperm count include:

- Serophene oral, however, is more normal in female nurses
- Gonal-F RFF Redi-ject (follitropin alfa or gonal-F)
- Antitoxins, if a low sperm count happens because of a urinary or conceptive lot disease
- Human chorionic gonadotrophin (Choragon or Pregnyl)
- Letrozole or anastrozole
- Exogenous androgens

Most exploration upholds the utilization of way-of-life changes, regular cures, and dietary changes to assist in further developodeveloperm the count.

Such way of life changes incorporate embracing an ordinary activity routine and rest plan, as well as keeping away from tobacco, overabundance of liquor, and illegal medications. It might likewise assist with keeping away from specific physician-endorsed meds.

Taking natural enhancements, like fenugreek and ashwagandha, may likewise help.

Dietary changes that advance a higher sperm count incorporate lessening the admission of trans unsaturated fats and expanding polyunsaturated unsaturated fat and vitamin D admission.

Keeping a restorative, adjusted diet that incorporates a lot of foods grown from the ground is the most ideal way to help sperm count through the eating regimen.

How does sperm motility influence richness?

Sperm motility is the capacity of sperm to proficiently move. This is significant in fruitfulness as sperm travel through the female regenerative plot to reach and prepare the egg. Low sperm motility can be a reason for male component barrenness.

What is sperm motility?

There are two sorts of sperm motility, alluding to how the singular sperm swims.

Moderate motility alludes to sperm that are swimming in a generally straight line or huge circles.

Non-moderate motility alludes to sperm that don't go in straight lines or that swim in extremely close circles.

For the sperm to overcome the cervical bodily fluid to treat a lady's egg, they need to have moderate motility of no less than 25 micrometers per second.

Unfortunate sperm motility or asthenozoospermia is analyzed when under 32% of the sperm can move effectively.

How can it influence ripeness?

Around the world, around 60 to 80 million couples are impacted by barrenness, and the rates fluctuate from one country to another.

In the US, the rate is believed to be associated with 10% of couples. The figure depends on the meaning of fruitlessness as the failure to consider following a year of endeavoring.

Male variable barrenness is the point at which an issue with the man's science makes him incapable of impregnating a lady. It represents between 40 to 50 percent of fruitlessness cases and influences around 7% of men.

Male fruitlessness is typically the consequence of a lack of information, the most widely recognized of which are:

- Low sperm count or oligospermia
- Unfortunate sperm motility
- Strange sperm shape or teratozoospermia

Around 90% of male barrenness issues are brought about by low sperm count, however unfortunate sperm motility is a significant element.

Reasons for low motility

The reasons for low sperm motility shift and many cases are unexplained.

Harm to the gonads, which make and store sperm, can influence the nature of sperm.

Normal reasons for gonad harm include:

- Contamination

- Testicular disease
- Testicular medical procedure
- An issue a man is brought into the world with
- Undescended gonads
- Injury

The drawn-out utilization of anabolic steroids can decrease sperm count and motility. Drugs, like pot and cocaine well as a few homegrown cures, can likewise influence semen quality.

Varicocele, a state of developed veins in the scrotum, has likewise been related to low sperm motility.

Semen examination is the most fundamental and helpful test, and it can recognize 9 out of 10 men with a ripeness issue. The test evaluates the arrangement of the sperm, as well as how they collaborate in the fundamental liquid.

The example is generally gathered by masturbation. The man will be approached to go without sex for somewhere in the range of 2 and 7 days before gathering the example to expand the volume of semen.

It is important for the entire discharge is be gathered in a sterile holder to guarantee the experimental outcomes are finished.

The example is normally gathered in a confidential room at the specialist's office or assortment office, however, even in certain conditions, it tends to be created at home. If so, the example should be conveyed for investigation soon.

The example ought not to be put away in the cooler, and specialists prescribe holding it near the body during transportation to keep it at an internal heat level. This will guarantee it is the most ideal quality when it is examined.

At times, the example can be gathered through sex, either in an extraordinarily planned condom or by pulling out before discharge. It is significant not to involve a business condom for this, as many have oils or spermicides that can pollute the example.

Tests can fluctuate for various reasons, including the length of restraint from sex and disease. Accordingly, two examples are typically gathered. They might be somewhere in the range of 2 to about a month separated.

On the off chance that the level of dynamically motile sperm is under 32%, the conclusion might be unfortunate sperm motility.

Instructions to further develop sperm motility

There is way of life decisions individuals can make that will assist with working on the nature of their sperm. Smoking can decrease ripeness and has been displayed to influence sperm motility.

Sporting medications, including weed, amphetamines, and narcotics, and extreme liquor utilization additionally lessen sperm quality. Specialists encourage individuals to stay away from these assuming that they are attempting to imagine.

Being overweight with a weight file of at least 25 can influence both the quality and amount of sperm.

There is a connection between an expanded temperature of the scrotum and a decrease in sperm. The ideal, sperm-creating temperature is around 94 °F, or just underneath internal heat level, so baggy clothing and going to basic lengths to keep the balls cool might help.

Supportive advances incorporate enjoying ordinary reprieves if working in a hot climate, and getting up and moving around on the off chance that an individual spends significant stretches plunking down.

There is no proof that correlative treatments are viable in further developing sperm motility.

Unfortunate sperm motility can prompt male fruitlessness, yet medicines are accessible. A few choices include:

Intrauterine insemination (IUI): Otherwise called planned impregnation, the IUI system includes sperm being gathered and washed. The quickest-moving sperm are then embedded into the belly utilizing a fine plastic cylinder.

In vitro preparation (IVF): During IVF, the lady is given medicine to empower the development of eggs, which are taken out from the ovaries and treated with sperm in the research facility. The subsequent incipient organism is then gotten back to the belly to create.

Sperm gift: An individual needing to imagine might have the option to get a sperm gift from a benefactor for use in an IVF technique.

Any individual who has been trying and failing to consider for over a year is encouraged to address their PCP to check for any ripeness issues there might be.

www.ingramcontent.com/pod-product-compliance
Lightning Source LLC
Chambersburg PA
CBHW060904260726
48661CB00008B/3451